Hernia

- a guidebook for patients and caretakers

Jacob Rosenberg, MD, DSc, FACS

ISBN-13: 978-1973850809
ISBN-10: 197385080X

Disclaimer

The information in this book is not intended as a substitute for the medical advice of a trained health care professional. You should consult a physician in matters relating to your health and any symptoms that may require medical attention.

Although the author has made every effort to ensure that the information in this book was correct at publication time, the author does not assume and hereby disclaim any liability to any party for any loss, damage, or lack of results associated with comments/text made by the author. This book is not intended as a substitute for the medical advice of physicians. The reader should regularly consult a physician in matters relating to his/her health and particularly with respect to any symptoms that may require diagnosis or medical attention.

Any information in this book should not be deemed as medical advice. You should not follow any potential advice in this book without checking with your own surgeon or other medical physician of your choice. The information in this book is best used to supplement your knowledge and expectations before or after consulting your surgeon or physician.

Hernia

a guidebook for patients and caretakers

Table of contents

Preface

There is no formal specialisation in hernia disease but I would nevertheless characterise myself as a hernia specialist. Hernia surgery constitutes the major part of my clinical as well as scientific work and it has had my interest for decades.

Numerous people around the World will experience a hernia during their lifetime and we all have friends or family members who have had hernia surgery. Being this common it is surprising that it is kind of low status within most surgical communities, and a hernia repair is often something that the youngest surgeon will do and consider it to be so-called "bread and butter surgery". This is definitely a wrong approach because hernia surgery is a surgical area, which is in fast development with new mesh materials and new operative procedures. Furthermore, our understanding of the biology of hernia formation is exploding in these years with exciting new data on genetic causes.

Being such a common disorder and such a common operative procedure it is surprising how little information is available for patients. This is the exact reason why I chose to write this short book oriented for the patient. The information within this book is not exclusively based on scientific evidence because in many areas the evidence is not adequate, but also derived from clinical practice, routines and traditions in most countries regarding diagnosis and management of hernia disease.

The book will not be a comprehensive textbook covering all areas of hernia disease but I have tried to cover the most important areas so that you, as a patient, hopefully will benefit from reading it.

Enjoy!

Introduction

I suppose that you have a hernia or that you know someone who has a hernia. Hernia disease is one of the most common conditions on the globe and hernia surgery is probably the most common surgical procedure performed worldwide. However, hernia is not a singular entity as it covers many different types of hernias with different clinical presentation, epidemiology, and management strategies. The most type of hernia is the inguinal hernia followed by umbilical hernia and then the more rare conditions.

I am sad to say that in many surgical departments an uncomplicated hernia is often repaired by the youngest surgeons in the department, but of course after adequate training and guidance by a more experienced colleague. This said, I would advise you to seek surgical care by someone with a specific interest in hernia disease as there are many new developments available in this clinical area, and by seeking a surgeon with a special interest in hernias you will probably receive up-to-date care and at least can be involved in the choice of different surgical approaches on a sound background.

However, do not be afraid if your operation will be performed by a young surgeon because it has been shown that the results of the operation is exactly as good if a young surgeon is performing the surgery as long as he or she is supervised thoroughly by a more experienced colleague. The essence is therefore that the surgical team is well educated and with an interest in hernia disease and management.

Hernia is gaining very much attention in these years with also formation of scientific societies and with high standards of clinical as well as scientific practice. It has been possible now to develop international guidelines for management of hernias, which is in fact extraordinary. This is not seen in many other clinical areas. The process of developing international guidelines is quite intense with years of hard work with participation of hernia surgeons from around the globe. You can find the link to the guidelines on the website given in the appendix.

Chapter 1:
General issues

The most common surgical condition in the world

Groin hernia is the most common surgical condition worldwide affecting around 27% of males and 3-4% of females. Groin hernia is divided in inguinal hernias and femoral hernias, with femoral hernias more often affecting women and inguinal hernias more often affecting men. However, men can also have a femoral hernia and women can of course also have an inguinal hernia.

The second most common condition is the umbilical hernia, which affects all age groups from newborns to the very elderly.

The epigastric hernia, also called linea alba hernia, is also a common condition and it is a bit more challenging surgically than the groin and umbilical hernias because of a high recurrence rate, i.e. that the hernia will come back despite good surgical technique.

The hernia type that is probably the most challenging for the surgeon as well as the patient is the incisional hernia. Unfortunately incisional hernias are quite common and they are more often seen after midline incisions than after transverse incisions. The reason why an incisional hernia can be challenging is that the recurrence rate is unfortunately quite high. This may be due to the basis of the disease meaning the reason why the patient developed the incisional hernia in the first place. It is probably caused by healing problems (intrinsic factors within the patient) and not so much by other factors. Although, if bad surgery has been performed with improper fascial closure, then the risk of developing an incisional hernia will of course be increased. This said, the most probable cause of an incisional hernia is the healing capacity of the patient.

There are other types of hernias as well and they include the sportsman's hernia, parastomal hernia, Spigelian hernia, lumbar hernia, perineal hernia, etc. They will be covered in a chapter by itself later in this book.

There is in fact a type of hernia that may

be more common than all the other hernias combined. This is the hiatus hernia where a part of the stomach is herniating through the diaphragm into the thoracic cavity. The reason why this is not normally considered formally a surgical condition is that most often the hernia is not repaired surgically and is treated pharmaceutically instead. The reason for this is that the main symptom of a hiatus hernia is acid reflux and this can in most cases be controlled by simple lifestyle or pharmacological measures.

The biology of hernia formation

Until recently is has been unclear why a primary hernia develops. We are all born with a natural umbilical hernia because the umbilical cord is passaging through the umbilicus from the baby to the placenta. This leaves a fascial defect after birth but in most babies this will close quite fast and most often within the first few years of living. Babies may also be born with an inguinal hernia because of lack of closure of the so-called processus vaginalis, which is left open after passage of the testicles from the abdomen where they are formed to the scrotum. The testicles are passaging through the inguinal canal and this "testicular highway" should normally be closed after the passage is over.

Most hernias, however, develop later in life and even though we are formed with intact fascia coverage of the abdominal cavity then the fascia may be disrupted at some point in life with the development of a primary hernia. The most typical primary hernias are hernias in the groin area, umbilical hernias and epigastric hernias.

The so-called secondary hernias are hernias after a previous surgical incision, so a secondary hernia is also called an incisional hernia. Having a surgical procedure for something else will create a fascial defect but normally the suturing of the fascia at the primary operation will be enough to secure good coverage of the abdominal content. In some cases, however, the closure is not adequate or it will create some weak spots that will later on develop into an incisional hernia.

Recently, it has been established that there is a certain inheritance pattern for inguinal hernias and the strongest tendency for the offspring to develop a hernia is in fact when a girl has a mother who has had a groin hernia.

Another recent exiting finding was the establishment of certain genes that apparently are coding for collagen formation and thereby theoretically for the risk of development of hernias. This does not in full explain the inheritance pattern of hernia disease so the area is probably more complexed than simple inheritance from father or mother to son or daughter. It may therefore be a disease involving multiple genetic loci and perhaps also environmental factors. This area is in fast development so hopefully in few years from now we will know much more.

It has also been established that hard labor is probably involved in the pathogenesis of especially lateral inguinal hernias in men when they appear later in life. It is reasonable to believe that hard labor also can be involved in the development of other types of hernias but these data are not available at the moment.

Watchful waiting

In many clinical areas it is good clinical practice to employ so-called watchful waiting. This means that the healthcare professional will advise you to wait a little and see if symptoms will get better or worse before an intervention is planned.

Within the area of hernia disease, however, this is probably not a good idea. A hernia will inevitably develop with time into a larger hernia and this means that the symptoms will get worse and especially the surgical management will be more difficult. "More difficult" means that the risk of complications will be increased so all together watchful waiting in hernia disease is not advisable unless the patient has severe comorbidities and therefore a very high risk of surgical complications.

Of course all hernias will not explode in size and symptoms with time and if life expectancy is not very long then it could be a good idea actually not to perform the operation and just wait and see if symptoms are sparse. In incisional hernias the outcome of surgery is unfortunately sometimes not optimal with a substantial risk of recurrence, so if symptoms are not impairing the social life of the patient then it could be discussed if watchful waiting would be an option in the individual patient situation.

Operation yes/no

There are many horror stories on the Internet about complications of hernia surgery, complications related to the mesh or the development of disabling chronic pain. This is both right and wrong because complications do occur but in surgical centers dedicated to hernia surgery the complication rate is low when the right patients are operated with the right techniques and by the right surgeons.

It is overall recommended to use a mesh for all types of hernia repairs other than in children. All groin hernias can be repaired with a mesh-based technique and using a mesh will enable the surgeon to perform the operation as so-called "tension free" meaning that the degree of pain after surgery is probably less and the risk of recurrence is also much less when looking at nationwide numbers. Thus, with the older suture-based techniques that we used before the Lichtenstein repair technique was introduced had a reoperation rate for recurrence around 20% when looking at national numbers. After introduction of the Lichtenstein technique, which is an open repair using a mesh in the groin, then the reoperation rate for recurrence is around 5-6% on a national level. It is very important, however, to underline that there are specialised surgical clinics available that use suture-based techniques and have exceptionally good results with very low recurrence and complication rates. This just emphasises the value of the surgeon.

The results in groin hernia repair after using a laparoscopic technique is even better with recurrence rates on a national level around 3-4%. Thus, the recurrence rate will probably be even lower at dedicated hernia centers.

The use of open pre-peritoneal techniques for groin hernia repair is gaining popularity and these techniques do have even lower complication and recurrence rates. This said, however, the use of these newer and specialised techniques are often employed by specialists with a scientific interest in a certain surgical technique so the reported very good results in the scientific papers may not be the same if the techniques are used throughout a nation. This is what we normally refer to as "external validity" so when you read a scientific paper for a special surgical procedure performed in a highly specialised unit and often by very few experienced surgeons then you can not automatically conclude that the results will be the same if the technique is spread to many different surgical departments.

We don't have sufficient data on pain after ventral hernia repairs (umbilical, epigastric and incisional hernias) but we do know something after groin hernia repair. There are numerous reports in the literature and from many countries around the globe that some patients will develop disabling chronic pain after open groin hernia repair using a mesh, the so-called Lichtenstein repair. The frequency of this serious complication is not fully elucidated because some reports have given numbers up to around 20% and others have given numbers in the vicinity of 1%. Many reports have not sufficiently distinguished between pain that are present, meaning that the patient has some kind of sensation in the groin after the procedure, to pain that is impairing daily activities for the patient. We know that young males may be a special risk group and patients with preoperative pain also have a higher tendency to develop pain after operation. Chronic pain is normally defined as pain lasting more than 6 months after operation. It is also known however, that pain will often fade away in the coming years and probably with a significant cut-off point around 3-4 years after operation. For most patients the long-term prognosis is therefore good but a small group of patients will still have problems years after surgery. These patients may be offered additional surgical procedures where the mesh is removed and a so-called triple neurectomy is performed. This means that the three major nerves innervating the groin area will be removed during the surgical procedure also with removal of the mesh. This has shown good results for chronic pain but of course the patient will develop numbness in the groin area when the nerves are removed.

You should not be alarmed by the information above because the choice of operation will always be a discussion between patient and surgeon taking lots of different factors into account. This mainly involves the degree of bother that the hernia has on the patient's daily life together with risk factors for complications after operation. A hernia will not disappear without surgery and will in most cases develop into a bigger problem with time. It is therefore in the vast majority of cases indicated to perform the operation and then when using a meticulous surgical technique and preferably a minimal invasive approach this will minimise the risk of severe complications after operation.

If you have access to surgical care in a highly specialised hernia clinic then it is absolutely okay to have an open repair without a mesh if this is the expertise of the clinic but for the majority of patients the choice does not involve this option and then my recommendation will be to have a laparoscopic or open pre-peritoneal repair if the surgeon masters one of these techniques. Laparoscopic groin hernia repair is gaining popularity in many countries and in my country it now constitutes around 50% of the procedures.

Length of convalescence after hernia repair

There are great variations between nations and even between different departments in the recommendations for length of convalescence. There are no scientific data to support a certain recommendation so whatever you hear from your surgeon it will be based on common sense and clinical experience.

If your hernia is repaired by a mesh-based technique then the healing mechanism after operation involves the ingrowth of connective tissue from your body into the mesh material. If the mesh is moving then the ingrowth will be impaired. This is probably the reason behind most surgeons recommending a few weeks absence from heavy workload and heavy sport activities. Normal daily clinical tasks such as walking and carrying a normal bag to and from a desk type job will most probably not impair healing and thereby not influence the risk of recurrence after the hernia repair. This is the reason why most surgeons will recommend only a few days convalescence after a non-complicated hernia repair and if you have a desk type job. If you have a job involving a heavy physical workload or if you are performing sport on an elite level then the recommendation for length of convalescence will probably be around 2-4 weeks depending on the type of activity.

Chapter 2:
Inguinal hernia

Definition

A groin hernia is a hernia in the groin area and they are divided into inguinal hernias and femoral hernias. An inguinal hernia is defined by the hernia defect that is placed above the inguinal ligament as opposed to the femoral hernia where the defect is placed below the inguinal ligament. There are two types of inguinal hernias, the medial hernia and the lateral hernia.

The lateral hernia is believed to be caused by an insufficient closure of the internal opening where the testicles have passed from the abdominal cavity through the inguinal canal to their placement in the scrotum during pregnancy. If this opening is not closed sufficiently then there will be a possibility for herniation.

The medial inguinal hernia is placed medially to the epigastric inferior vessels (as opposed to the lateral hernia where the hernia defect is placed laterally to these vessels). The defect in the transversalis fascia and muscle layers is placed in the back wall of the inguinal canal. The abdominal content (the bowel and/or fat) can then pass through the hernia defect directly into the inguinal canal area and the patient will see and feel an inguinal bulge.

It is practically impossible to distinguish between a lateral and a medial inguinal hernia before operation.

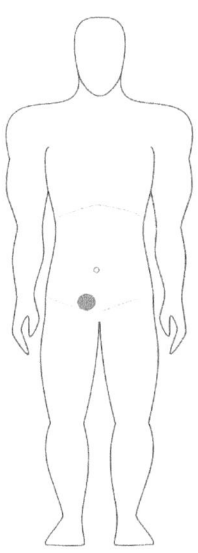

Risk factors

Recent data have shown that hard physical labor is probably a risk factor for the development of symptomatic lateral herniation. This association between labor and herniation is not present for medial hernias.

It is also known that the occurrence of inguinal hernia is much more common in men than in women although the inheritance pattern is stronger for women than men. The exact explanation for this epidemiology of hernia disease is presently unknown.

It has also been shown that the presence of certain genes can predispose to the development of hernia and we are awaiting further data in this very interesting clinical area in the coming years.

Around 27% of all men on the globe irrespective of race will develop an inguinal hernia during their lifetime. It is therefore one of the most common diseases worldwide.

Symptoms

The clinical symptoms of an inguinal hernia are ranging from almost nothing to only cosmetic complaints through to severe pain and social disability because of the hernia. If the lump is big or painful then sexual activity may also be impaired because of the hernia. The hernia may be small and only present during heavy coughing or physical strain or it may be large going from the inguinal area down to the scrotum and may be difficult to reduce in some cases.

It is important that the hernia can be reduced because an incarcerated hernia may potentially have impaired blood supply (called strangulation) and thereby risk of tissue ischemia and subsequently necrosis. However, if you have a reducible hernia then the risk of incarceration is very low so there is no need to worry about this during your daily activities. On the other hand, if it is irreducible and if pain develops it may be a sign of strangulation and you need to seek medical advice immediately.

Treatment – open repair

The most common treatment of an inguinal hernia worldwide is the Lichtenstein procedure which is an open anterior repair where a mesh is placed with a tension free technique. The mesh is fixed to the tissue typically by sutures but it can also be fixed by staples or glue. The open repairs can be divided into the open sutured repairs, the open repairs with placement of a mesh, and the open pre-peritoneal mesh repairs.

The open sutured repairs are the oldest operative techniques for repair of an inguinal hernia. Many different techniques have been available for decades and the best known of these techniques today is the Shouldice repair that is used in few clinics around the world and with good results. When I say good results, I mean low recurrence rates and low incidences of chronic pain. It seems, however, that the Shouldice repair requires surgical technical training at a level that is not performed in many standard university clinics around the world. It is therefore a good operation for a dedicated hernia clinic that has specialised in this particular technique. During a Shouldice repair the back wall of the inguinal canal is repaired by layers of sutures and thereby the hernia defect is closed and the inguinal area is strengthened.

The open anterior mesh repairs are now almost exclusively performed by the so-called Lichtenstein technique which was invented by Dr. Lichtenstein in the US. With this technique, a polypropylene (or polyester) based mesh is placed covering the back wall of the inguinal canal and thereby strengthening this area also with a narrowing or closure of the hernia defect during the procedure. In the Lichtenstein repair it is possible to strengthen the abdominal wall without pulling on the muscle and fascia structures causing tension and thereby a theoretical risk of pain and recurrence. Furthermore, the Lichtenstein technique is quite easy to teach young surgeons and therefore it gained wide spread popularity around the globe within very few years. For the last 30 years or so it has been the most popular operative technique for repair of inguinal hernia. However, there are also potential problems. Reports started to come out that chronic pain was an issue although the recurrence rates decreased from previous open sutured repairs (typically the so-called Bassini and McVay techniques) from around 20% down to around 5%. Thus, the positive result was that the recurrence rate decreased dramatically after introduction of the Lichtenstein technique; but the occurrence of chronic pain seems to be higher than with the previous techniques. It should be emphasised, however, that we actually do not have reliable data from the old sutured repair techniques regarding chronic pain so it is impossible to give an honest answer whether the rates of chronic pain actually increased with the introduction of the Lichtenstein technique or if it now was just studied in more detail. When placing a mesh in this position with the Lichtenstein technique then the mesh will be placed in very close vicinity to some of the nerves in this region. In some patients the obligatory slight shrinkage of the mesh after the operation will sometimes entrap a nerve and thereby probably contribute to the development of chronic pain. The pathogenesis of chronic pain is however multifactorial so this hypothesis is just one of many. Rarely a mesh infection can occur and this is treated by removal of the mesh and surgical drainage. However, this is a rare phenomenon occurring in less than 1% of operations in most clinics.

The new kid on the block in open repairs are the techniques where the mesh is placed behind the back wall of the inguinal canal, thus at the same position as with the laparoscopic repair (see below). With the open pre-peritoneal mesh repair the skin is incised in the inguinal region and the mesh is pushed through an opening in the back wall of the inguinal canal and then placed in the pre-peritoneal space. The advantage of this approach is that the risk of chronic complaints and chronic pain seems to be substantially lower than when placing the mesh in front of the back wall of the inguinal canal. Behind the back wall there are not nerves present to the same extent as in front of the back wall in the inguinal area, and this is probably the main reason why results are encouraging for the open pre-peritoneal mesh based techniques. These operations are in development presently and if you search for information you should look for operations like the TIP, TREPP, TRIP, or the ONSTEP techniques. Not all clinics can offer these techniques and as for any surgical approach there is a degree of specialisation to take into account. This means that the clinic you are approaching will most probably have a preference for surgical approach and it gives good meaning to accept this preference because it means that they have good quality for the approach that they have chosen to use in most cases.

Treatment – laparoscopic repair

Laparoscopic repair for inguinal hernia can be performed by two different techniques the so called TEP repair and the TAPP repair. The abbreviations stand for Totally Extra Peritoneal repair (TEP) and Trans Abdominal Pre-Peritoneal repair (TAPP). There is no difference in clinical outcome with the two techniques meaning that the recurrence rates and rates of chronic pain are comparable for the TEP vs. the TAPP. Therefore, as mentioned above, the preference of the clinic that you are approaching is the correct choice because they have gained routine and good clinical quality with their chosen technique.

With the TEP technique three incisions are made in the midline below the umbilicus. One incision is made for the camera port and then there are two incisions for small trocars that will hold the dissecting instruments. The instruments are not passing through the peritoneum into the abdominal cavity but is placed extra-peritoneally, thereby the name TEP. The inguinal area is dissected in that the peritoneum is pushed away from the structures from the inguinal area. It is then possible to reduce the hernia sack no matter if it is a lateral hernia, a medial hernia or a femoral hernia. The dissection technique is the same for all three hernia types where the peritoneum is separated from the vessels and muscle structures in the inguinal region. Thereafter, a polypropylene (or polyester) based mesh in the size of 10x15 cm is placed covering all potential hernia defects, i.e. a lateral defect, a medial defect and a femoral defect. The mesh will cover all potential defects and thereby the risk for a new hernia is probably diminished. The mesh is often not fixed to the structures because it will be held in place when the instruments are removed and peritoneum is covering the area. Some surgeons will use mesh fixation with either titanium clips, titanium tacks or absorbable tacks. It is also possible to fixate the mesh by fibrin sealant glue or by artificial glue like cyanoacrylate or similar.

The TAPP technique is a little different from the TEP technique. With the TAPP technique the trocars and instruments are pushed through the abdominal wall into the abdominal cavity and the operation is performed from inside the abdominal cavity into the inguinal region. The peritoneum is incised and the dissection is thereafter somewhat similar to the TEP dissection where the peritoneum is separated from the vessels and muscular structures in the inguinal region. After the dissection and the reduction of the hernia sack a 10x15 cm polypropylene (or polyester) based mesh is placed covering all potential hernia defects in the region. With the TAPP technique it is most common to fixate the mesh and the typical fixation technique is by tacks, either permanent (titanium) or absorbable tacks. There are good results with glue fixation but this is not performed in all clinics. After the mesh is fixated the peritoneum is closed and the closure of the peritoneum has to be sealed either by suturing, tacking or gluing peritoneum together.

Chapter 3:
Femoral hernia

Definition

A femoral hernia is protrusion of abdominal content below the inguinal ligament. This is opposed to the inguinal hernia, where the hernia bulge is placed above the inguinal ligament. The hernia defect is always placed at the same position in a femoral hernia, and that is medial to the femoral vein, which is the large vein draining blood from the leg. Under the inguinal ligament the femoral vein, the femoral artery and the femoral nerve are passing from and to the leg. If there is extra space medial to the femoral vein, then a herniation is possible.

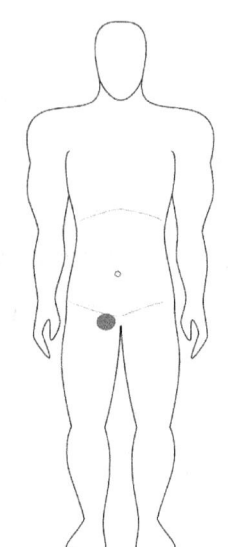

Risk factors

Femoral hernia is more common in women than in men. The reason for this is probably the often wider pelvis in females compared with males. When the pelvis is wider, then there will be more space below the inguinal ligament and medial to the femoral vein, and therefore making development of a femoral hernia possible. Nevertheless, men can certainly also have a femoral hernia but it is just more common in females.

Symptoms

The symptoms of a femoral hernia are often more subtle than the typical symptoms from an inguinal hernia. The reason for this difference in clinical manifestation is unknown but it is known to all surgeons that a femoral hernia may present itself with a sudden bowel obstruction although the hernia bulge may have been present on and off for years in the same patient. Often the fatty tissue in the area of the femoral hernia is large enough in a female that it may be difficult to discover that a hernia is present until it gives serious symptoms from strangulation or incarceration.

Treatment – open repair

A femoral hernia may be operated by open technique which years ago was typically by the McVay technique, where the muscle plate with the transversalis fascia was sutured to the fibrous structures covering the pubic bone. This operation has been replaced by the mesh-based open technique, which is a slight modification of the traditional Lichtenstein technique (see description under inguinal hernia). Thus, when operating a femoral hernia by open technique with a mesh then the polypropylene (or polyester) based mesh is sutured in a way that it covers the back wall of the inguinal canal, and then it is fastened to the fibrous structures covering the pubic bone and exactly lateral to the hernia defect the mesh would be sutured to the tissue covering the femoral vein and artery.

Treatment – laparoscopic repair

It is recommended that all femoral hernias are repaired by laparoscopic technique because of a lower recurrence rate and probably also because it is easier to perform the operation by laparoscopy than by open technique for most surgeons confident with laparoscopic repair. When femoral hernia is much more common in females than in males, then in practical terms it means that a woman with a hernia in the groin area will be offered laparoscopic repair as a routine in most departments around the world.

The operative technique for laparoscopic repair of a femoral hernia resembles the technique for laparoscopic repair of an inguinal hernia whether it is TEP or TAPP technique. The operation is performed by separating the peritoneum from the structures in the groin area (vessels, muscles and fat etc.) and then placing a 10 x 15 cm polypropylene (or polyester) based mesh that covers all the possible hernia defects i.e. the femoral hernia defect and also a potential medial and lateral defect. At the end of the mesh placement peritoneum is in the TAPP technique closed by either tacks, clips, sutures or glue, and in the TEP technique the instruments are simply withdrawn and the peritoneum will cover the mesh.

Chapter 4:
Umbilical hernia

Definition

An umbilical hernia is a hernia that passes through the umbilicus through a fascia defect. The hernia comes in all sizes from the tiniest hernia which is maybe a few millimeters to large herniations like a basketball in extreme cases. An umbilical hernia is a primary hernia meaning that operation has not been performed in the area before.

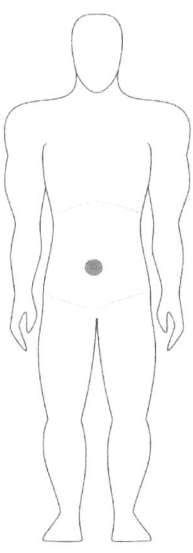

Risk factors

It is unknown whether an umbilical hernia is more likely to occur if the patient has hard physical labor. It is well-known, however, that pregnancy will predispose to the development of an umbilical hernia and some medical diseases can also cause umbilical hernia, e.g. severe liver disease with fluid in the abdominal cavity (ascites). Umbilical hernia is obligatory in the newborn because of the umbilical cord passing through the umbilicus. In most babies, the defect will close very fast and a hernia will not develop clinically. In some children, an umbilical hernia will develop but as the defect will close in about 90% before the age of 3 years it is advised that surgical repair is postponed until the child is about 3 years old.

Symptoms

The symptoms of an umbilical hernia are often pain and cosmetic complaints. The bulge in the umbilical area is easily seen even when wearing clothes so the cosmetic indication is certainly a clinical scenario. An umbilical hernia will in many patients also cause pain and if the hernia is incarcerated or even strangulated then the pain will of course be acutely worsened. If the hernia is strangulated then acute surgical intervention is indicated.

Treatment – open repair

The most common surgical procedure for umbilical hernia is simple open repair where the hernia defect is sutured. Until recently it was often sutured with absorbable suture material but is seems that this will produce a high recurrence rate so most surgeons have now changed to non-absorbable sutures for primary closure of the umbilical hernia defect. Nevertheless, even with meticulous surgical technique and proper suturing of the defect with non-absorbable suture the recurrence rate may still be as high as 20%.

There is therefore currently a development where after closure of the fascia with non-absorbable suture a polypropylene or polyester based mesh may be placed with an onlay technique meaning that the mesh is secured to the fascia on top of the sutured hernia defect. It is also possible to place the mesh below the fascia and then close the fascia on top of the mesh. These techniques have published results regarding recurrence rate that are much better than the simple sutured repairs but still recurrence rates around 10% have been reported with the mesh-based technique for open repair. It has also been shown that even when placing a mesh for the repair, the rate of chronic complaints will not increase compared with the simple sutured repair. It therefore seems reasonable to move in the direction of mesh-based repair techniques for umbilical hernia and we are awaiting the development in the coming years.

Treatment – laparoscopic repair

An umbilical hernia may also be treated by laparoscopic technique and with good results. With the laparoscopic technique, a covered mesh is placed intra-abdominally covering the umbilical hernia defect. There is a current development ongoing where many surgeons will close the hernia defect laparoscopically (meaning from the inside) before placing the mesh on the previous hernia defect. The results with defect closure before mesh placement are promising, but the general opinion is that we need more data before it can be recommended for all umbilical hernia repairs.

A mesh based on polypropylene or polyester has to be covered by other material because it is in contact with the bowels. This will inhibit ingrowth of bowels into the mesh. The mesh has to be secured to the peritoneum and transversalis fascia from inside and this mesh fixation can be done by different methods including permanent tacks, absorbable tacks and sutures. It can also be a combination of these different fixation techniques. The mesh may also be fastened by glue instead of tacks or sutures but there was a high recurrence rate when only using glue from mesh fixation. There are also data available pointing at absorbable tacks as the only fixation technique to be insufficient in that the recurrence rate may be significantly higher than when using permanent fixation with tacks and/or sutures.

For the laparoscopic repair 3 small incisions are made in the left side of the patient's abdomen and through these 3 small incisions a camera port and 2 trocars for working instruments are introduced into the abdominal cavity. The hernia content is then dissected and placed in the abdomen and the hernia defect is in some surgical centers closed by sutures. Then the mesh is introduced into the abdomen and placed on the hernia defect and fastened by tacks and/or sutures.

The procedure is typically done in an outpatient basis even with the laparoscopic repair under general anesthesia.

Chapter 5:
Epigastric hernia

Definition

An epigastric hernia is also called a linea alba hernia and is placed in the midline between the umbilicus and sternum.

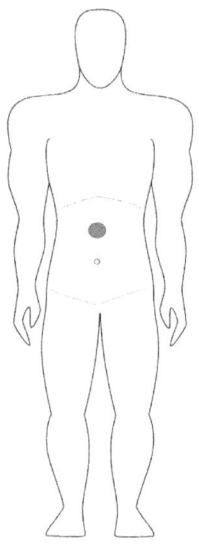

Risk factors

There are no known risk factors for the development of an epigastric hernia. It is sometimes seen in patients who also have other hernias so perhaps some kind of genetic disposition is present, although it has not been shown scientifically. Moreover, there are no data to support a connection between hard physical labor and the development of an epigastric hernia.

Symptoms

An epigastric hernia most often gives distinct symptoms for the patient. If the hernia defect is small then symptoms are often pain because of incarceration of the herniated tissue. If the hernia defect is large then the symptoms often comprise complaints from the large bulging including cosmetic complaints as well as pain.

Treatment – open repair

An epigastric hernia can be repaired by open surgical technique where a transverse incision is placed on top of the hernia. The hernia is then dissected from the surrounding fatty tissue and the hernia content is placed intra-abdominally. The fascia defect is then closed by sutures which nowadays are most often non-absorbable for this indication. Many surgeons will reinforce the abdominal wall in the hernia area by placing a small piece of polypropylene or polyester based mesh on top of the fascia after closing the defect with non-absorbable sutures. It may also be possible to place the mesh below the fascia and then close the fascia on top of the mesh.

Treatment – laparoscopic repair

An epigastric hernia may be repaired by laparoscopic technique and the surgical technique is more or less the same as for laparoscopic repair of an umbilical hernia. The operative steps therefore include placement of 3 trocars in the left side of the patient's abdomen, dissection of the hernia content and placing it in the abdominal cavity. Some surgeons will then close the defect by laparoscopic suturing and some will just place a mesh on the area (from inside of course) covering the hernia defect. If the hernia defect is sutured then a mesh will also be placed on the hernia defect. The mesh has to be fixated and this is done by tacks and/ or sutures. Since the mesh is in contact with the bowels it has to be a special type of mesh with a covering membrane that will inhibit ingrowth of bowel into the mesh.

Chapter 6:
Incisional hernia

Definition

An incisional hernia is a hernia through an abdominal wall defect placed in a previous surgical incision. An incisional hernia is therefore also called a secondary hernia opposed to the primary hernias that occur without a previous operation in the same place. An incisional hernia may occur all over the abdomen in previous incisions.

Risk factors

There are known risk factors for the development of an incisional hernia. The best described risk factors are the occurrence of a wound infection at the primary operation and especially if there has been wound dehiscence after the primary surgical procedure. Another risk factor is smoking, meaning that if the patient is smoking when having the primary operation then the risk of developing an incisional hernia is increased. Lastly, there is some evidence available pointing at genetic predisposition with impaired collagen formation as a possible risk factor for the development of an incisional hernia. It has also been established that if the primary operation was performed through a vertical incision compared with a transverse incision then the risk of developing an incisional hernia is increased.

Symptoms

The symptoms of an incisional hernia resembles the symptoms of the other hernias on the front abdominal wall. Thus, the symptoms may involve cosmetic complaints, bulging and pain. Incarceration and strangulation of an incisional hernia is a quite rare phenomenon so the operation is most often performed as a planned procedure instead of an acute intervention.

Treatment – open repair

Treatment may be performed by various open repair techniques but all the techniques used today involve the use of a mesh. Without a mesh, the risk of recurrence is substantial so a mesh is recommended for all repairs of incisional hernias. One of the problems with the open repair techniques is that it often involves quite extensive dissection and thereby the risk of mesh infection and wound infection is increased. If at all possible many surgeons therefore tend to choose a laparoscopic repair because of the low risk of infectious complications. Open repair is recommended for the smallest incisional hernias as well as for the larger hernias whereas the mid-size hernias tend to be operated more by laparoscopic technique. The reason why the largest incisional hernias are operated by open technique is that they often involve special procedures on the abdominal wall muscles in order to get coverage of the hernia defect. Some of these procedures cannot be performed by laparoscopy and an open approach is therefore recommended. The sizes preferred for open technique will in many departments be the hernia defects below 2-3 cm and above 10 cm in diameter. The group with hernia defects between around 2-3 cm up to 10 cm are in many places offered a laparoscopic repair if the surgical expertise is available locally.

Treatment – laparoscopic repair

Laparoscopic repair of an incisional hernia is performed technically in the same way as laparoscopic repair of umbilical and epigastric hernias. In the incisional hernia, however, there are often intra-abdominal adhesions because of the previous surgical procedure and therefore it may take longer time to perform the procedure and it does involve some risk of bowel lesion because of the adhesiolysis before a mesh can be placed covering the hernia defect. The choice between open and laparoscopic repair and especially the choice in the first place whether the hernia should be operated or not is something that the patient and the surgeon will discuss together. It is most often advisable to follow the surgeon's recommendation of technique because the choice of operative approach of course also depends on the local expertise and traditions. This means that if local expertise is especially high for a certain operative approach, then the complication rates for this technique at this specific surgical center is probably lower than when using other techniques at that particular center.

Chapter 7:
Other hernias

Sportsman's hernia

A sportsman's hernia is a strange condition because it is actually not a hernia. A hernia is defined as the protrusion of intraabdominal content through the abdominal wall and a sportsman's hernia does not involve a defect in the abdominal wall.

It is a clinical condition where typically a physically active person (that is why it is called a sportsman's hernia) can develop symptoms in the groin that resembles symptoms of a groin hernia. It is, however, not possible to find an abdominal wall defect with a herniation in such a patient.

There a numerous hypotheses around why a physically active person can develop groin pain and the most reasonable explanation is that hard physical strain on the groin area can cause tendinitis in some of the tendon or fascia structures in the area. This is most typically in the medial part of the groin where maximum pain point will be on the bony structures and the adjacent fibrous tissue. This can easily be provoked by simple physical examination where the surgeon will press these fibrous structures in the medial part of the groin and this will normally produce quite severe pain in a patient with a sportsman's hernia. If at the same time there is not at formal hernia present then the diagnosis is clear.

The condition can be treated by various techniques. Most important is of course to stop what caused the condition in the first place and that is why it is recommended to decrease physical activity that has caused the pain. This is of course impossible if the patient is for instance a professional football player so other means have to be chosen.

There are good results from some clinics with repeated blockades by injecting local anesthetics and/or steroids in the fibrous tissue where maximum pain is present. However, in some cases this therapeutic approach is not sufficient.

Various operative techniques have been

used where some have divided the painfull tendon structures and others have performed a regular hernia repair although there has not been a hernia present at all. It seems, from the literature, that the best results from surgical intervention are obtained by performing a laparoscopic inguinal operation with placement of a mesh fixated by fibrin sealant or glue. The reason why placing the mesh is actually helping on the pain in such a condition is to be honest unknown. Perhaps the placement of a mesh and performing an operation will keep the patient from performing strenuous physical activity for period of time and that may be the reason but it may also be something absolutely different. Nevertheless, it seems to work in many patients so if conservative treatment (no physical activity with standard anti-inflammatory pain killers) does not work and if repeated injected blockades does not work then a laparoscopic placement of a mesh in the groin area may be the way to go.

Parastomal hernia

Unfortunately, many patients develop a parastomal hernia after an intestinal stoma has been created. This is seen both in small bowel as well as large bowel stomas. Some reports have mentioned numbers up to 50% of patients developing a parastomal hernia and some have given even higher numbers. A parastomal hernia may be very bothering for the patient because it may make it quite difficult to fit the stoma dressings and sometimes it will produce leaks from the stoma bag as well as of course pain and other complaints. In a parastomal hernia the opening in the abdominal wall is widening so that bowel and fatty tissue from the abdomen will pass through the abdominal wall and lie in the subcutaneous tissue under the skin level around the stoma itself. That is why a bulge is seen in the stoma area in these patients. It may be quite difficult to reduce the hernia and a typical situation is that the bulging is a permanent situation in these patients with difficulties in fitting the stoma dressings etc.

Until recently the typical repair technique would be to perform a new laparotomy and move the stoma to the other side of the abdomen and close the abdominal wall where the hernia was present. This is indeed major surgery and therefore it is not a good option in all patients.

In recent years various mesh based repair techniques have been described and the most successful techniques are probably the laparoscopic approach with placement of a mesh to cover the defect in the abdominal wall around the bowel passing through the muscle layers. Nevertheless, there may be complications involved in these laparoscopic procedures because there will be sometimes quite extensive dissection in an area with adhesions after previous operations. This will increase the risk of bowel lesions during the hernia repair and a bowel lesion will often make placement of a mesh impossible because of risk of infection. There are, however, numerous reports available of successful laparoscopic management of parastomal hernias so if the surgeon is confident that this will be a good option for you then it would be the way to go.

The best approach, however, will be to avoid the hernia occurring in the first place. Prevention of parastomal hernia seems to be possible by placing a mesh at the primary operation where the stoma is created. If a mesh is placed during that operation then the risk of developing a parastomal hernia is almost avoided in many of the published series. This technique is slowly gaining popularity around the globe and many departments are now changing their clinical routines and will in the coming years more and more use mesh placement around the stoma at the primary operation. Therefore, hopefully, we will see less stomal hernias in the coming years.

Spigelian hernia

A Spigelian hernia is a rare condition where abdominal content is herniating through part of the abdominal wall and it is placed along the lateral edge of the rectus muscle. It can occur all the way from caudal to cranial on the abdomen but always along the lateral edge of the rectus muscle. A Spigelian hernia is usually quite small and the diagnosis may be difficult because the hernia is not palpable superficially meaning right under the skin as other hernias are but the hernia sack may only pass through some of the abdominal wall layers and not all of them. This combined with the typical patient having a few centimeters of fatty tissue under the skin will make normal clinical diagnosis difficult. Often, a patient will have an ultrasound scan to show the hernia dynamically meaning with and without coughing or pushing abdominal content out through the hernia defect. It is difficult to perform such a dynamic diagnostic test with a CT or MRI scans and that is why ultrasound scan is the best option here. Very often, simple clinical examination is sufficient to give the diagnosis. These hernias are passing through typically a quite small hernia defect and that is why they often give severe pain symptoms.

It may be difficult to repair a Spigelian hernia by open technique because when the hernia sack is passing through only some of the levels of the abdominal wall and often not in a direct line from the abdomen to the outside (see figure) then an open approach may be quite difficult in some patients. It is therefore easier to perform the operation by laparoscopic technique and during the laparoscopy it is typical to see a very small slit in the peritoneum and this is where the intra-abdominal content passes through the abdominal wall layers and gives symptoms for the patient. During the laparoscopic operation the slit may be simply covered by an onlay mesh, which is covered on the inside where it touches the bowels. It may also be a good option to take down the peritoneum and by this remove the hernia sack an then place a polypropylene mesh behind the peritoneum, thus not touching the bowels and the peritoneum is thereafter closed covering the mesh. This technique is the preferred surgical option and with published very good results.

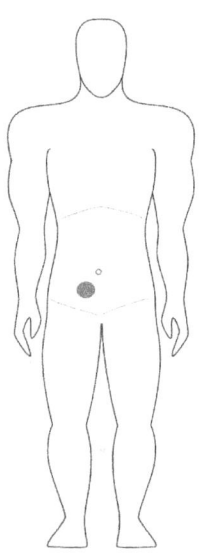

Perineal hernia

A perineal hernia is a rare condition and may be caused by complicated vaginal delivery, trauma, or after surgical intervention in the area.

The perineum is the area between the anal opening and the scrotum in men or the vagina in women. This area is normally covered by a thick muscle layer as well as fascial covering. If a vaginal delivery has been extremely complicated with rupture of the pelvic floor then a perineal defect may be the long-term result. It may also be caused by trauma to the region or may be seen after some of the newer operative techniques for low rectal cancer. During these operations, a quite large area is excised in order to remove the malignant tissue and this will in some cases leave a perineal defect even though it is closed initially during the operation.

Treatment of a perineal hernia is challenging and the results from external repair by suturing the defect is not optimal with risk of recurrence. It may be associated with infectious complications to place a mesh in open repair because of the vicinity to the anal opening. This is why repair from the inside (by laparoscopy or open surgery) may be preferable but this will be technically difficult because of the narrow pelvis where dissection, suturing and mesh placement is obviously not an easy task. Recently, use of the robot for these types of operations have gained some popularity and probably with good reason since it is easier to manoeuvre in the small pelvis using the robot assisted laparoscopic technique compared with classical laparoscopy or open intraabdominal repair. Only few centers around the world have extensive experience with these procedures.

Hiatus hernia

A hiatus hernia is a sliding herniation of the upper part of the stomach into the thoracic cavity (see figure)

This condition will in most cases not be offered surgical repair because the symptoms which are mainly in the form of gastroesophageal reflux disease (GERD) can most often be handled by medical therapy. This will not cure the disease but it will alleviate the symptoms and therefore surgical repair is not the primary option.

If medical treatment is failing then surgical repair may be a good option. The surgical procedure is a fundoplication where the stomach is withdrawn to the abdomen and then the fundus part (the upper part) of the stomach is wrapped around the lower esophagus, and the opening in the diaphragm is narrowed by a few sutures in the diaphragm muscle. The procedure is laparoscopic with very short hospitalisation and in many centers it is performed on an outpatient basis.

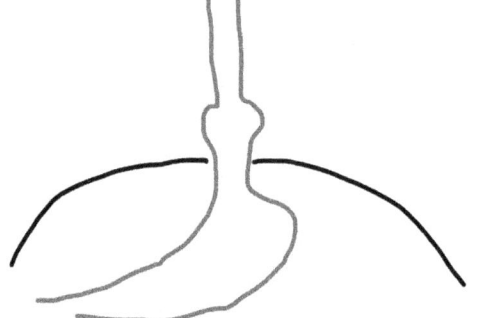

Paraesophageal hernia

A paraesophageal hernia is like the sliding hiatus hernia also a herniation through the diaphragm but in the paraesophageal hernia the esophagus and stomach is not sliding into the thoracic cavity but typically only the fundus (upper) part of the stomach is herniating along the esophagus and thereby the name paraesophageal (see figure). In this situation the pressure on the content that is passing through the defect in the diaphragm is typically high and may therefore produce a significant risk of tissue ischemia in the herniated part of the stomach.

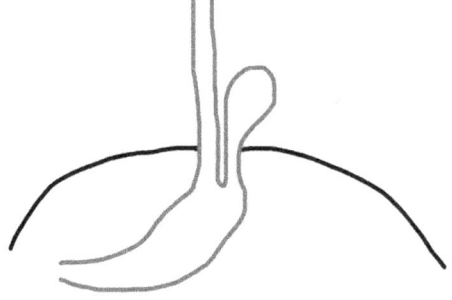

As the herniation is inside the body a lump or bulge is not seen on the outside. The diagnosis is therefore often difficult and the symptoms vary. Typical symptoms would be symptoms from the cardiopulmonary system with breathing difficulties, asthma, palpitations, episodes with tachycardia, and many more. This complex clinical presentation often results in late diagnosis and patients have typically been to many different specialists before the diagnosis is finally made.

It is easy to establish the diagnosis using

oral contrast radiology where the patient drinks a contrast solution and at the same time simple x-rays or a CT scan are performed.

Treatment is surgical and in most patients an operation is indicated because of the risk of tissue ischemia in the herniated part of the stomach. If this tissue becomes necrotic then the mortality is high. It is therefore recommended to perform an operation in most patient.

There are different operative approaches for a paraesophageal hernia but all of them will of course include reducing the hernia meaning removing the herniated part of the stomach from the thoracic cavity and placing it in the abdomen. In the abdomen then some kind of procedure is needed to avoid the herniation from reoccurring. Many surgeons prefer to perform a fundoplication just as in the sliding hiatus hernia in order to keep the stomach inside the abdomen. This can be performed with or without a mesh to cover the enlarged hiatus (the natural defect in the diaphragm where the esophagus is passing from thorax to the abdomen). It may also be an option to do a so-called gastropexy where the stomach is sutured to the front abdominal wall and thereby kept in the abdomen rather than making it possible to slide back into the thoracic cavity.

Pediatric inguinal hernia

Inguinal hernia may be seen in the newborn as well in the elderly. In small children an inguinal hernia is considered to be more dangerous than in the adult. The reason for this is probably that a child does not have intraabdominal fatty tissue so a herniation in a child is almost always bowel compared to an adult where the herniated tissue is very often intraabdominal fat. This is probably the reason why it is recommended to perform surgical repair in all children with an inguinal hernia. An inguinal hernia defect in a child will not close without surgical intervention and that is why surgical repair is indicated (in contrast to the pediatric umbilical hernia where surgical repair is not routinely recommended before the age of 3 because of natural closure of the hernia defect in most children).

In the very small children, probably up to 2-3 years of age, then the inguinal canal is not fully developed so the repair technique is different than when performing pediatric inguinal hernia repair in a larger child. A newborn does not have an inguinal canal and the hernia sack is therefore protruded directly from the abdomen through a defect and into the palpable bulge under the skin. When the child is growing the natural defects in the abdominal wall will slide where the most profound defect will slide laterally and the superficial defect will stay medially. This will form the inguinal canal that is present in the larger child and of course in all adults.

In the newborn, the repair technique therefore involves only excision of the hernia sack and not closure of the defect because the defect will in the next few years naturally slide and form the inguinal canal. In the larger child (approximately 3-10 years) and the adolescent (11-18 years), the repair technique is different and will be a suture repair where the defect is located and sutured so that the herniation will be prevented. It is not normal practice to use mesh material in patients under 18 years old.

However, some adolescents are already physically big when presenting with an inguinal hernia, and if they are considered fully grown it may be indicated to insert a mesh for the repair. This issue is debated among hernia specialists and there are no current guidelines for the management of inguinal hernia in this age group.

Some centers are experienced in laparoscopic repair of pediatric inguinal hernia and with this technique the defect is located by laparoscopy and is narrowed by simple suturing during the procedure.

Pediatric umbilical hernia

All babies are born with an umbilical defect because of the umbilical cord. This umbilical defect will in most babies close very fast but in some it will persist. If a small child has a persisting defect then an umbilical hernia will be seen.

As there is almost no intraabdominal fat in a small child then the herniated tissue will almost always be bowel and that is why attention is given to all children with hernias. However, it is seen in about 90% of all small children with an umbilical hernia that the hernia defect will naturally close without surgery up to the age about 3 years. This is why the usual recommendation is to wait until the child is about 3 years of age and then if the hernia still persists a surgical repair is performed. Surgical repair in a 3-year old will be a simple suture repair since mesh insertion is not recommended for children below 18 years of age.

Chapter 8:
FAQ

What is a hernia?

A hernia is the protrusion of abdominal content through the abdominal wall making a visible bulge. Most hernias are visible of the front abdominal wall and they include inguinal hernia, femoral hernia, umbilical hernia, epigastric hernia, Spigelian hernia, and incisional hernia. There may also be a kind of "internal" herniation where part of the stomach is herniating through a defect in the diaphragm from the abdominal to the thoracic cavity. This is called a hiatus hernia or a paraesophageal hernia. They are still hernias even though the bulge is not visible from outside.

Is there a risk of a new hernia developing at the same side of a previous hernia repair?

This is called a recurrence and although many surgical procedures for hernia are safe and with very good results there are no techniques available with 0% recurrence rate.

Can a hernia cause urological problems?

If an inguinal hernia is large, then it may sometimes make it difficult for the patient to urinate because of simple pressure to the penis and urethral areas. After hernia repair when this pressure is removed the urinating function will most likely be normalised. However, it is well known that an inguinal hernia repair, especially by open technique under epidural or spinal anesthesia, may cause urinary dysfunction with urinary retention and the need for catheterisation and subsequent prostatic surgery. The reason for this has not been fully elucidated but is probably due to subclinical prostatic disease that becomes visible with clinical symptoms when the patient has had either spinal or epidural anesthesia. This is the main reason why epidural or spinal anesthesia (so called regional anesthesia) is not advised for open hernia repair as a general rule. These urination problems are not seen to the same extend after operation under local infiltration anesthesia or under general anesthesia.

Will my hernia repair cause sexual dysfunction?

It has been shown that some patients will develop sexually related pain after especially open repair of an inguinal hernia. The rates of sexual dysfunction after surgery are varying in different publications so the exact frequency is not known. On the other hand, quite a few patients who experienced sexual dysfunction before hernia surgery will actually experience improvement after the inguinal hernia has been repaired. The reason for this may be that the bulge in the groin area will physically impair sexual function because of contact-related pain during intercourse.

Can my hernia be repaired on an outpatient basis?

Most hernias can be repaired in an ambulatory setting without formal hospitalisation. Only the largest incisional hernias and other types of ventral hernias may sometimes require hospitalisation for a few days, especially because of postoperative pain or if a surgery related complication occurs.

How long will my convalescence period be?
There are two types of convalescence, the time to return to normal daily activities and the time to return to work. Time to return to normal daily activities is from a medical point of view not limited. The hernia procedure should be sufficient enough to enable the patient to return to normal daily or leisure activities as soon as he or she wants to do that. Time to return to work is a bit more differentiated as it depends on the type of work that the patient has. If the patient has a desk-job then he or she can return to work already a few days after the surgical procedure. If work is strenuous then a longer sick leave is recommended by most surgeons. The length of the sick leave is based on traditions more than on scientific data. Most surgeons nowadays will probably recommend a sick leave around 1-2 weeks if the patient has medium to hard labor and 3-4 weeks if the job

type is physically very demanding. The same goes for recommendations for when the patient can perform sporting activities. Most sporting activities are physically hard work, so a general recommendation of a convalescence period from sporting activities of around 3-4 weeks is used by many surgeons. It should be emphasised, however, that there are no data whatsoever to support a certain length of convalescence so the given numbers are from common sense and traditions more than from science.

Is there a risk of significant blood loss during hernia surgery?

The simple answer is definitely no. The average blood loss for a hernia repair is probably around 3-5 ml and only in rare cases bleeding is more than this. This is also the reason why preoperative blood reservation is not indicated on a routine basis.

What is the difference between a reducible,

an incarcerated and a strangulated hernia?
A reducible hernia can be pushed back into the abdomen. Most hernias are reducible and they can therefore be repaired as a planned surgical procedure. An incarcerated hernia is defined as a non-reducible hernia and an incarcerated hernia may sometimes be operated semi-electively meaning that the patient should not wait for several months to undergo surgery. However, some patients may have had an incarcerated hernia for years and in such a clinical scenario surgical repair can be performed as a planned procedure without urgency at all. If the hernia gets strangulated it means that the incarcerated hernia now has some additional symptoms. The most common symptom in this setting is the development of pain and if an incarcerated hernia is becoming painful, then it is by definition strangulated until proven otherwise. This means, that a painful incarcerated hernia should undergo emergency repair, because there is a risk of impaired tissue blood supply and thereby an

increased risk of severe complications without urgent surgery.

Will my hernia go away without treatment?
No hernia will disappear without surgical repair. The only exceptions are the pediatric umbilical hernia in children below 3 years and the adult sportsman's hernia (but that is actually not a hernia - see the book section about sportsman's hernia). Thus, a sportsman's hernia may sometimes disappear with either medical therapy, physiotherapy or repeated injected blockades but all other hernias will require surgery to disappear.

Is it dangerous to have a hernia?
As a general rule it is not dangerous to have a hernia. The risk of strangulation is very small so the indication for surgical repair is in the majority of cases the complaints such as pain or discomfort from the hernia. Having said this, it should be emphasised that in some patients the hernia will increase in size with time making it

surgically more difficult to repair the hernia defect without risk of complications.

How physically active may I be after a hernia repair?

As a general rule the surgeon may tell you that you can do whatever you want but it should not hurt. If you experience pain in the surgical area after operation, then you should of course stop the activity that you are doing and wait a while until you can do it without pain.

I had a groin hernia repair, but there is still a bulge?

After groin hernia surgery some patients will experience a bulge where the hernia was present preoperatively. This may be due to a seroma which is a fluid collection in the previous hernia cavity. This will disappear with time, but it can take several months before it has fully disappeared. A seroma may also occur after the other hernia repair types but it should in most cases be managed conservatively meaning that it should not be drained, because with drainage there is a risk of infection. It will disappear in almost all patients after some months.

What is the risk of recurrence after an inguinal hernia repair?

This question is a bit difficult to answer because most publications have not been able to follow their patients after the operation with a 100% follow-up. However, a recent publication (American Journal of Surgery 2016;212:391-398) has given some interesting results. They showed that a direct inguinal hernia (also called a medial hernia) was associated with an increased risk of recurrence compared to an indirect (lateral) hernia. Current smoking was also an independent predictor of recurrence as well as old age. Nevertheless, there is absolutely no reason to be alarmed because the overall recurrence rate in this publication was only 0.8%. This must be due to short or suboptimal follow-up because data from the Danish National Hernia Database have shown recurrence rates on a national level around 5% after inguinal hernia repair.

Why do I need a mesh for my hernia repair?
The main reason why most surgeons have changed surgical routines and now uses mesh for inguinal hernia repair is because of the recurrence rate. Before we used a mesh on a routine basis, sutured repairs (without a mesh) showed recurrence rates around 20%. After the introduction of a mesh whether it is used for the open Lichtenstein repair or the laparoscopic repair the recurrence rates have decreased dramatically and in many centers it is as low as 1-2% and on a national level it is probably around 5%. However, there are clinics that have specialised in sutured repair without a mesh and they show remarkably low recurrence rates for their patients. It may therefore also be a matter of focus and surgical technique where the use of sutured repair without a mesh can produce good results with almost no recurrences.

Overall, for the average surgical clinic the results with using a mesh is definitely better regarding recurrence rates compared with a sutured repair without a mesh.

When can I go to the fitness center or go for a run after my hernia repair?

The answer to this question is not based on scientific evidence. There are no data available to give a definite answer so we have to rely on common sense and traditions, unfortunately. Most surgeons will tell you to wait with sporting activities for a few weeks after the operation, typically around 2-4 weeks. However, you can return to normal daily activities already on the day after the operation, meaning that you can go for a walk or even carry your bag and groceries. You should not go home and lie on the sofa because then you actually will increase your risk of complications related to inactivity. It is therefore a good idea to return to your normal daily activities as soon as possible.

Should I choose a laparoscopic or an open repair?

The recommendation is that you should choose whatever your surgeon recommends. The reason for this is that the surgeon will recommend the type of surgery that he or she is most confident in. Thereby you will receive the type of surgery with the best results in the particular setting. When we overall look at data on e.g. a national level, the results seem to be better with laparoscopic compared with open repair. However, if your surgeon has better results with open repair, then this is absolutely the way to go. The choice of surgical technique should therefore be taken in collaboration between the patient and the surgeon.

What is a sports hernia?

A sports hernia is also called a sportsman's hernia and it is actually not a hernia. A hernia is when there is a distinct defect in the abdominal wall with protrusion of intra-abdominal content as a bulge under the skin. A sportsman's hernia is not a hernia because there is no bulge. It is a symptom complex caused by inflammatory changes in the fibrous tissue where some of the muscles are fastened to the bony structures in the inguinal area. The typical place of the inflammation and pain is in the medial part of the groin where some of the tendons and muscles meet the pelvis bone. If the surgeon puts pressure on these points there will be a distinct pain. The diagnosis can also be visualised with ultrasound examination where there will be local tissue oedema and reaction corresponding to the area with intense pain. Treatment is primarily conservative with anti-inflammatory drugs, physiotherapy, and/or repeated injected blockades. If this does not help, then surgery may be indicated.

What tests are needed to diagnose a hernia?
In most cases the diagnosis is quite easy and can be done by simple physical examination. The surgeon will examine you with his or her

fingers and maybe ask you to cough while standing up and then palpate the groin area at the same time. This will in the majority of cases give the diagnosis. Sometimes diagnosis may be difficult, especially with increased body weight and fatty tissue in the area. If the surgeon is in doubt of whether there is a hernia or not, then he or she may send you to an ultrasound scan or in some rare cases even to a CT-scan. The latter is more often used for incisional hernias where a CT-scan can determine reliably the size of the defect in the abdominal wall and thereby the operation may be planned better before surgery. In most cases, however, the diagnosis is straight forward and is only confirmed by simple clinical examination.

Do I risk losing a testicle if I have hernia surgery?

About 30 years ago this was part of the preoperative information to patients before open inguinal hernia repair. Fortunately, time has changed. Nowadays the risk of losing a testicle during surgery is close to 0%. In my many years of practice I have never seen it happen. There is though a slight risk of so-called ischemic orchitis with subsequent testicular atrophy after inguinal hernia repair. This is still a very rare phenomenon. Some patients will experience testicular pain for a period after operation and in some of these patients the testis may reduce its size with time. The reason is probably a decreased blood flow to the testicle after surgery. As mentioned this is extremely rare in daily clinical practice, but the risk is not 0%. Some reports have shown about 2% risk of testicular pain with subsequent reduced testicular size. It is, however, based on old data and my impression is that it does almost not occur nowadays.

Hernias during pregnancy
If you develop a hernia during your pregnancy then the overall recommendation is to wait and see. It is not dangerous to have a hernia during

your pregnancy but it may in some cases be associated with complications for yourself or the baby if you have hernia surgery during pregnancy. If the hernia gets strangulated then of course you should have acute surgery. Elective repair, however, can be postponed to some months after the pregnancy.

Can I prevent myself from getting a hernia?
The simple answer is no. A hernia does not develop because of your behaviour so relax and simply see a surgeon to get advice for a repair. You may think that a certain physical activity provoked the formation of the hernia because it became apparent after for instance a run or after heavy lifting. It may have been timely correlated to a certain event, but the hernia only came out because there was a weakness in the abdominal wall corresponding to the placement of the hernia so at some point you would have gotten the hernia anyway. Therefore, do not blame yourself since the hernia would most probably have become apparent with or without

your physical activity.

Are hernias hereditary?

This is in fact a complicated question because we have only recently found a few genes that seem to code for impaired collagen formation and the development of hernias. The results are new and we do not at this point exactly know the clinical meaning of these findings. It is nevertheless an area of intense research so hopefully in a few years we may be able to answer the question. It has been shown, however, that there is a distinct family pattern for some families with an increased risk of the children getting a hernia if the parents have had a hernia.

Chapter 9:
Closing

Closing remarks

Congratulations that you have made it to the end of this book. I hope that you have found the information that you needed and will approach your surgical hernia repair with confidence and without fear. This was the main aim of the book and although it is obvious that it has not been possible to cover all areas of hernia disease and hernia repair in a book like this, I hope that the information provided has been sufficient. If you need specific other information than given in the book please feel free to write me an email and I will include it in an upcoming edition of the book.

Contact information

jacob.rosenberg@regionh.dk

About the author

Jacob Rosenberg (1964) was born and grew up in Copenhagen, Denmark. He is professor of surgery at the University of Copenhagen, and chief surgeon at the Gastro-unit, surgical section, Herlev Hospital (also in Copenhagen).

The author page at amazon.com is: https://www.amazon.com/author/ jacobrosenberg

Appendix

American Hernia Society:
americanherniasociety.org

European Hernia Society:
europeanherniasociety.eu

Asia Pacific Hernia Society:
aphernia.org

British Hernia Society:
britishherniasociety.org

Hernia Society of India:
hsi-aphs.com

Canadian Hernia Society:
canadianherniasociety.ca/en/

World Guidelines for Groin Hernia
Management:

ehs2016.eu/images/content/overig/
herniasurgeguidelinesstatementsrecommendatio
ns.pdf

Notes

Notes